HANDBOOK OF PRACTICAL PHYSICAL PHARMACEUTICS FOR B.PHARM STUDENTS

Jasmine kaur Randhawa

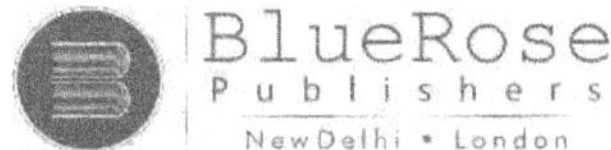

BlueRose
Publishers
NewDelhi • London

First Published in October 2021

ISBN: 978-93-5472-553-1

BLUEROSE PUBLISHERS

www.bluerosepublishers.com

info@bluerosepublishers.com

+91 8882 898 898

Cover Design:

Mukti Verma

Typographic Design:

Ilma Mirza

Distributed by: BlueRose, Amazon, Flipkart

DEDICATED

TO

MY MOTHER

Acknowledgements

I am greatly thankful to my family for support during the compilation and preparation of the manuscript.

My special thanks to the team of Bluerose publications for the help and encouragement given to me during the preparation of this book.

Jasmine kaur Randhawa

2 September 2021

PREFACE

Physical pharmaceutics is a subject concerned with physical science aspects of pharmaceutics. The practical physical pharmaceutics deals with the practice of physical aspects of pharmaceutics. The problem is that very few books are available that deal with practical physical pharmaceutics as compared to theory books. So effort is made to cover the practicals needed to be performed during B.Pharm curriculum. This book will be very helpful for the teachers and students dealing with pharmacy education. This book is written in simple english and in a precise way to overcome any difficulty in studies. This book consists of 20 practicals with special emphasis on practical aspects of topics like viscosity, surface tension, density, particle size, pH, stability of suspensions , etc.

Suggestions and criticism are welcomed from the teachers and students.

Tarn Taran

2 September 2021   **Jasmine kaur Randhawa**

INDEX

AIM: To study the effect of concentration of liquid on viscosity

REFERENCE: Subrahmanyam C.V.S, Textbook of physical pharmaceutics, Vallabh parkashan, 2007: 236-243

APPARATUS: Beaker (250 ml), measuring cylinder (100ml), pipette (50ml), rubber tubing, stop watch, thermometer (100°C,Ostwald's viscometer, volumetric flask (200ml & 100ml), water bath

CHEMICALS REQUIRED: Sucrose, purified water

THEORY: Viscosity is an index of resistance of a liquid to flow. The higher the viscosity, the greater is the resistance to flow. Viscosity is calculated by the following formula:

$$\eta = F/G$$

Coefficient of viscosity is defined as the force per unit area required to maintain unit difference in velocity between two parallel layers in the liquid, one centimeter apart. It is expressed as centipoises cp(=0.01 poise)Poise is defined as the shearing force(stress) required to produce a velocity of 1cm/sec between two parallel planes of liquid each 1 cm square in area and separated by a distance of 1 cm. Viscosity is influenced by two type of factors:

1. Intrinsic factors

2. Extrinsic factors

Intrinsic factors: chemical nature i.e., molecular size, shape and intermolecular forces, influence the viscosity.

Extrinsic factors: Pressure, temperature and additives influence the viscosity. Added substances such as small quantities of nonelectrolytes like sucrose , glycerine and alcohol when added to water, the solution exhibits increased viscosity.

PROCEDURE:

Prepare sucrose solution A by transferring accurately weighed 22.2 gm of sucrose into a 200ml volumetric flask and make up the volume upto the mark with water to prepare the solution with concentration of 111mg/ml.

Transfer 100 ml of 'solution A' to a 200 ml volumetric flask and make upto the mark with water with mixing to prepare solution B.

Transfer 100ml of solution B to a 200 ml volumetric flask and make the volume upto the mark while mixing to prepare solution C.

1. Fill the clean and dried viscometer with sucrose solution A using the pipette.
2. Gently clamp the viscometer in the water bath maintained at temperature 37°C.
3. Fit the rubber tubing to one end of viscometer and gently blow to push the level of the solution above mark E.
4. Stop blowing, allow the liquid to fall from mark E and measure the time taken using a stop watch and record.
8. Empty the viscometer and rinse with few aliquots of the solution B.
9.Repeat the steps 4 to 7 using the solution B.
10. Empty the viscometer and rinse with a few aliquots of the solution C and repeat the steps 4 to 7 using the solution C.
11. Empty the viscometer and rinse with water.
12. Repeat the steps 4 to 7 with water.
13. Determine the kinematic viscosity 'v' for each solution using the following formula:-

$$V = kt$$

Where v=kinematic viscosity in area covered per second (mm^2s^{-1})

$\quad$ K= viscometer constant=$0.003mm^2s^{-2}$

$\quad$ t= time in seconds(s)

Observations:-

Solution	Kinematic viscosity(v)
A	
B	
C	
Purified Water	

Calculate the sugar concentration (mg/ml) for each solution

Solution	Concentration(mg/ml)
A	
B	
C	
Purified Water	

Plot a graph of kinematic viscosity (y) against concentration(x)

RESULT: The viscosity of water increases/decreases with increase in concentration of sucrose.

AIM: To determine the viscosity of given liquid by using ostwald's viscometer at room temperature.

REFERENCE: Subrahmanyam C.V.S, Textbook of physical pharmaceutics, Vallabh parkashan, 2007, 257-261

APPARATUS: Ostwald's viscometer, pipette, stopwatch, rubber tubing, beaker, burette stand

CHEMICALS REQUIRED:-Given liquid, purified water

THEORY: Ostwald's viscometer is a single point capillary viscometer used to determine the viscosity of a Newtonian liquid.

The viscosity of the given liquid using the following equation

$$\eta_1 = \frac{\rho_1 t_1}{\rho_2 t_2} \eta_2$$

Where ρ_1= density of the unknown liquid

t_1= time of flow of unknown liquid

ρ_2= density of the known liquid at room temperature

t_2= time of flow of known liquid(water)

η_2= viscosity of the known liquid (water) i.e. 1.01 centipoises

η_1 = viscosity of given unknown liquid

Ostwald's viscometer is used to determine the kinematic viscosity of liquids.

Applications: Ostwald viscometer is used for quality control purposes in the formulation and evaluation of pharmaceutical dispersion systems such as colloids , dilute suspensions, emulsions, etc. It is official in IP for the evaluation of liquid paraffin and dextran 40 injection (plasma expanders).The study of flow of liquids through a capillary tube throw light upon circulation of the blood.

PROCEDURE:

1. Select a clean and dried Ostwald's viscometer and fix firmly to a stand in vertical position.
2. Transfer a fixed amount of water through a wide limb with the help of a pipette.
3. Using a rubber tube, blow to push the level of water above the upper mark A.
4. Allow the water to flow down and when water meniscus reaches the mark A , start the stop clock.
5. Stop the stop clock when water meniscus reaches the mark B.
6. Note the difference in time which represents the flow of time for a given liquid water.
7. Rinse the viscometer with the given test liquid and repeat the steps 2-6 for the given liquid.
8. Calculate the viscosity of the given liquid using the following equation

$$\eta_1 = \frac{\rho_1 t_1}{\rho_2 t_2} \eta_2$$

Where ρ_1 = density of the unknown liquid

t_1 = time of flow of unknown liquid

ρ_2 = density of the known liquid at room temperature

t_2 = time of flow of known liquid (water)

η_2 = viscosity of the known liquid (water) i.e. 1.01 centipoises

η_1 = viscosity of given unknown liquid

RESULT: The viscosity of given liquid sample is ....centipoises.

AIM: To study the viscosity of given sample by using Brookfield viscometer.

REFERENCE: Subrahmanyam C.V.S., Textbook of physical pharmaceutics, Vallabh parkashan, 2007, 388-389

APPARATUS: Brookfield viscometer, beaker, calibrated thermometer, water bath capable of maintaining required temperature

THEORY: Brookfield viscometer mounted on helipath stand with T spindle is ideal to study the behaviour of settling of suspensions. The T bar rotates and changes its position continuously .At the same time , it also descends slowly into the liquid sample with the help of synchronous motor .The path traced by the spindle is helix. As the T bar moves , the liquid offers resistance. The dial reading indicates the magnitude of resistance. Thus using T spindle and helipath , the dial reading can be plotted against the number of turns of spindle.

PROCEDURE:

1. Confirm that the viscometer has been calibrated
2. Confirm that the viscometer is leveled using the bubble level on the back of the instrument.
3. Equilibrate the temperature of the sample liquid to the temperature designated in the specification
4. Auto zero the instrument with no spindle attached and speed set as designated in the product specification. The main display will flash 00.0 after 10 seconds.
5. Attach the selected spindle to the on the spindle shaft of the viscometer. Transfer the given sample into a beaker and dip the spindle into the sample. Do not allow air bubbles to be formed. The spindle should not touch the bottom or sides of the container and should be centered. Reconfirm that the viscometer is leveled properly.
6. Choose the units by pressing the desired unit key(CPS for centipoises)

7. Set the desired speed (rpm) ,start the viscometer by pressing the key motor and read at constant reading.

8. When done, turn the motor and power off.

9. Clean the spindle and place in spindle holder.

10. If the low light comes on, the reading is approximate and indicate that the speed/spindle combination is not optimized(less than 10 % of full scale).Change the speed until the light goes off. Note the speed used .If the speed cannot correct the problem, change the spindle. Note the speed used. If the speed cannot correct the problem, change the spindle. Note the spindle used. For special projects, note temperature , spindle and speed used.

If EEE is displayed, the reading is over range, correct as given in 9.

RESULT: The viscosity of given liquid sample is ....centipoises.

AIM : To determine the surface tension of given liquid using stalagmometer

REFERENCE: Subrahmanyam C.V.S., Textbook of physical pharmaceutics, Vallabh parkashan, 2007, 129-135

APPARATUS: Stalagmometer, rubber stopper, a small piece of rubber tube, a screw pinch cork, beaker.

THEORY: Surface tension is defined as the force, in dynes, acting on the surface of the liquid at right angles to any line of length of surface,1 centimeter. The units of surface tension are dyne/cm in CGS system and Newton/meter in MKS system. Surface tension is an important physicochemical property and a characteristic of a liquid. Some liquids posses higher surface tension.

The surface tension of the given liquid using the following formula:

$$Y_2 = \frac{n_1 d_2}{n_2 d_1} \times Y_1$$

Where n_1 = number of drops of water between mark A and B.

n_2 = number of drops of given liquid

d_1 = density of water at room temperature

d_2 = density of given liquid at room temperature

Y_1 = surface tension of water (71.6dyne/cm)

Y_2 = surface tension of given liquid

PROCEDURE:

1. Take a clean stalagmometer and rinse it with distilled water and then with ether

2. Attach a small rubber tube having a screw pinch cork to the upper end of the stalagmometer.

3. Fill it with water by immersing the lower end into distilled water and sucking the water above mark A.

4. Allow the water to fall down and count the number of drops obtained from a volume of water between the marks A and B.

5. Rinse the stalagmometer with the given liquid and then fill it with the given test liquid above mark A.

6. Count the number of drops for the volume of liquid between the marks A and B.

7. Calculate the surface tension of the given liquid using the following formula:

$$Y_2 = \frac{n_1 d_2 \times Y_1}{n_2 d_1}$$

Where n_1= number of drops of water between mark A and B.

n_2= number of drops of given liquid

d_1 = density of water at room temperature

d_2= density of given liquid at room temperature

Y_1= surface tension of water (71.6dyne/cm)

Y_2= surface tension of given liquid

RESULT: The surface tension of given liquid sample is ....N/m.

AIM: To determine the bulk and tapped density of given powder material

REFERENCE: Subrahmanyam C.V.S., Textbook of physical pharmaceutics, Vallabh parkashan, 2007, 215-216,226

APPARATUS: Bulk density apparatus, graduated measuring cylinder, weighing balance

CHEMICALS: given powder material (starch, lactose etc),

THEORY: Bulk density is mathematically defined as:

$$\text{Bulk density } (\rho) = \text{mass of the powder (w)/bulk volume(Vb)}$$

When particles are packed loosely, lots of gaps between particles are observed. Hence bulk volume increases making the powder light. Based on bulk volume, the powders are classified as light and heavy. Light powders have high bulk volume. On the other hand, smaller particles may sift between the larger particles, the powder assume low bulk volume or high bulk density. Such powders are known as heavy powders. The bulk density depends on particle size distribution, shape and cohesiveness of particles. Bulk density is used to check the uniformity of bulk chemicals (quality control measures).The size of capsule is mainly determined by bulk volume for a given dose of material. The higher the bulk volume (low bulk density) and bigger will be the size of capsule. Bulk density helps in selection of proper size of a container, packing material, mixing apparatus in the production of tablets and capsules. The capacity of a mixing bowl is usually expressed in cubic feet. Normally the volume of formulation and an excess of 10 % of the volume is considered for the selection of container for the mixing process.

Capacity of mixing bowl = weight of batch/bulk density

Tapped density is defined as the ratio of mass of powder to the tapped volume. Tapped volume is the volume occupied by the same mass of powder after a standard tapping of a measure. It is measured by the help of bulk density apparatus. The working of this apparatus is explained in the procedure given below.

PROCEDURE:

Pass the given powder material through a standard sieve No.20

1.   Note the weight of empty 100ml graduated cylinder. Let the weight be W_1gm
2.   Introduce the given powder material into the measuring cylinder and reweigh it. Let the weight be W_2gm.calculate the weight of powder material $W_3=W_2-W_1$gm
3.   Note the volume of material. Let it be V_1ml.
4.   Calculate the bulk density of material using the following formula:-
          Bulk density=W_3/v_1gm/ml
5.   Fix the cylinder containing powder material on the bulk density apparatus.
6.   Continue the tappings until a constant volume of powder material is obtained.
7.   Note the final volume. Let it be V_2ml.
8.   Calculate the tapped density using the following formula:-
          Tapped density=W_3/v_2gm/ml

RESULT: The bulk density of given powder sample is ....g/ml and tapped density is ....g/ml.

AIM: To determine the angle of repose of given powder material

REFERENCE: Subrahmanyam C.V.S., Textbook of physical pharmaceutics, Vallabh parkashan, 2007, 222-224

APPARATUS: Glass funnel, ring stand, ruler, weighing balance, protactor, pencil, paper

CHEMICALS: given powder material.

THEORY: The flow properties of a powder are measured by angle of repose .Improper flow of powder is due to the frictional forces between the particles. These frictional forces are quantified by angle of repose. It is defined as the maximum angle possible between the surface of a pile of the powder and the horizontal plane (surface). It is expressed as:

$$\tan\theta = h/r$$

$$\theta = \tan^{-1} h/r$$

Where h = height of pile formed

r = radius of the pile circle

θ = angle of repose

The lower the angle of repose, the better the flow property. Rough and irregular surface of particles gives higher angle of repose. Decrease in particle size leads to a higher angle of repose. Lubricants at low concentration decrease the angle of repose. Fines (passed through 100 mesh) increase the angle of repose. The procedure for measuring angle of repose of powder is explained below.

PROCEDURE:

1. Fix a glass funnel in place with a glass funnel in place with a clamp on a ring stand.

2. Transfer the powder material (after passing through a 10 mesh sieve) into the funnel and allow the powder to fall on a paper.
3. Maintain a 6.4mm gap between the bottom of the funnel stem and the top of the pile.
4. Measure the height of the pile (h) with the ruler.
5. Draw a circular line with pencil around the heap of the powder on the paper.
6. Measure the radius of the circle with the formula:-

$$\tan \theta = h/r$$

$$\theta = \tan^{-1} h/r$$

Relation between angle of repose and powder flow

Angle of repose(^{0})	Flow
<25^0	Excellent
25^0-30^0	Good
30^0-40^0	Passable
>40^0	Very poor

Result: The angle of repose of given powder is ....^{0} hence the type of flow of given powder is ....

AIM: To study the effect of glidant on flow properties of given powder

---

REFERENCE: Subrahmanyam C.V.S., Textbook of physical pharmaceutics, Vallabh parkashan, 2007, 222-223

APPARATUS: Glass funnel, ring stand, ruler, paper, tray, spatula, given powder, pencil, weighing balance

CHEMICALS: powder material, glidant (talcum, magnesium stearate)

THEORY: Same as experiment no. 6

The flow properties of a powder can be improved by incorporating optimum concentration of glidants such as magnesium stearate, talcum, etc. It is observed that glidants at lower concentration decrease the angle of repose and at higher concentration enhance the angle of repose.

PROCEDURE:

1. Fix a glass funnel on a ring stand and hold a paper below the glass funnel.
2. Transfer the powder material (after passing through a 10 mesh screen) into the funnel and allow the powder to fall on the paper below the funnel.
3. Maintain a 6.4 mm gap between the bottom of the funnel stem and the top of the pile.
4. Measure the height of the pile (h) with the ruler.
5. Draw a circular line with pencil around the heap of the powder on the paper.
6. Measure the radius of the circle formed with the ruler.
7. Estimate the angle of repose using the following formula:-

$$\tan \theta = h/r$$
$$\theta = \tan^{-1} h/r$$

8. Then add 5 % (5 gm in 100gm) of talcum in the powdered material in a tray.
9. Repeat the steps 1-7 for the powdered material mixed with glidant.

10. Calculate the angle of repose and study the effect of glidant on angle of repose

Observations:

Sample	Angle of repose($^\circ$)
Powder material	
Powder material with 5 % glidant	

Result: The angle of repose increases/decreases with the addition of glidant.

AIM: To determine the compressibility index of given powder

REFERENCE: Subrahmanyam C.V.S., Textbook of physical pharmaceutics, Vallabh parkashan, 2007, 226-227

APPARATUS: Bulk density apparatus, graduated measuring cylinder, weighing balance

CHEMICALS: given powder material

THEORY: The compressibility index is defined as:

Compressibility index=Tapped density-fluff density×100

Tapped density

It is indirectly related to the relative flow rate, cohesiveness and particle size. It is simple, fast and popular method of predicting powder flow characteristics.

Fluff density is the ratio of mass of powder to the fluff volume. Fluff volume is the volume occupied by a certain mass of powder when poured into the measuring cylinder.

Tapped density is the ratio of mass of powder to the tapped volume. Tapped volume is the volume occupied by the same mass of powder after a standard tapping of a measure.

The compressibility index can be a measure of the potential strength that a powder could built up in its arch in a hopper and also the ease with which such arch could be broken.

PROCEDURE:

1. Transfer a weighed quantity (about 20 gm) of the given powder into the graduated measuring cylinder
2. Note the initial volume occupied by the powder. Let it be V_0.
3. Calculate the fluff (poured) density of the powder using the following formula.

$$\text{Fluff (poured) density} = \frac{\text{weight of powder}}{V_0} \text{ gm/ml}$$

4. Then fix the measuring cylinder on the tapping apparatus and tap the contents until a constant volume is obtained.
5. Note the final volume of the powder. Let it be V_1 ml.
6. Calculate the tapped density of the powder using the formula:

$$\text{Tapped density} = w/V_1 \text{ gm/ml}$$

7. Calculate the compressibility index using the formula:-

$$\text{Compressibility index} = \frac{\text{Tapped density - fluff density}}{\text{Tapped density}} \times 100$$

Relation between compressibility index and type of flow

Compressibility index	Flow
5-15	Excellent
12-16	Good
18-21	Fair to passable
23-35	Poor
33-38	Very poor
>40	Very very poor

Result:-The compressibility index of given powder is ....

hence the type of flow is.................

AIM: To determine the particle size distribution of powder by sieving method.

REFERENCE: Subramanyam C.V.S., Textbook of physical pharmaceutics, Vallabh parkashan,2007,199-201

APPARATUS: Mechanical shaker apparatus, standard sieves of different mesh numbers, weighing balance

CHEMICALS: given powder material.

THEORY: Particles having size range between 50 and 150 µm are estimated using sieving method. In this method, the size is expressed as d sieve, which describes the diameter of a sphere that passes through the sieve aperture as the asymmetric particle. This method directly gives weight distribution. The sieving method finds application in dosage form development of tablets and capsules. Normally 15 % of fine powder (passed through 100 mesh) should be present in granulated material to get the proper flow of material and achieve good compaction in tabletting. Therefore, percent of coarse or fine powder can be quickly estimated. Sieves for pharmaceutical testing are constructed from wire cloth with square meshes, woven from wire of brass, bronze, stainless steel or any other suitable material. Sieves should not be coated or plated. There must be no reaction between the material of the sieve and substance to be sieved. Sieving method is inexpensive , simple and rapid with reproducible results.

PROCEDURE:

1. Select standard sieves of different mesh numbers
2. Arrange the sieves in a nest with the coarsest at the top.
3. Weigh about 50 gm of sample and place on the top sieve and fix the sieves set to the mechanical shaker apparatus and shake for a certain period of time(20minutes)
4. Weigh the powder retained in each sieve. Frequently ,the powder is assigned the mesh number of the screen through which it passes or on which it is retained .It is

expressed in term of airthmatic or geometric mean of the two sieves. For example, a powder passing through a 36 mesh and retained on 44 mesh sieve is assigned an arithmetic mean diameter of (425+325/2 or 375µm.This size is reported as undersize.

Observations:-

Sieve number(passed/retained)	Arithmetic mean size of opening(µm)	Weight retained on a sieve(gm)	Percent weight retained(undersize)	Cumulative percent weight retained

Analyse the above data for normal,log-normal ,cumulative %frequency distribution and probability curves.

RESULT: The size distribution of given powder material is from ....to .... µm.

AIM: To determine the particle size distribution by optical microscopy method.

REFERENCE: Subrahmanyam C.V.S., Textbook of physical pharmaceutics, Vallabh parkashan, 2007, 195-198

APPARATUS: Microscope, eye-piece micrometer

CHEMICALS: paraffin oil (liquid paraffin), given powder

THEORY: Particle size in the range of 0.2-100µm can be measured by optical microscopy. In this method, the size is expressed as dp (projected diameter), which describes the diameter of a sphere having the same area as the asymmetric particle when observed under a microscope. This method directly gives number distribution, which can be further converted to weight distribution. The optical microscope has a limited resolving power of the lens. The lower limit can be brought down using ultramicroscope and electron microscope. Optical microscopy is used to determine:

1) particle size analysis in suspensions

2) globule size distribution in emulsions

3) particle size analysis in aerosols

PROCEDURE:

1. Fitted the eye-piece of the microscope with a micrometer.
2. Calibrate the eye-piece micrometer using a standard stage micrometer.
3. Take the powder sample and prepare a suspension with a suitable vehicle such as paraffin oil (liquid paraffin).
4. Mount the suspension on a slide and place it on the mechanical stage.
5. Estimate the size of the particle with the help of the eye-piece micrometer.
6. Count around 625 particles in order to estimate the true mean.

7. Plot the size distribution curves such as normal, log normal, cumulative frequency and probability curves.

Mean size(μm) d	Log mean size Log d	% number of particles in each n	Cumulative % frequency number distribution	%frequency weight distribution(undersize)	Cumulative %frequency weight distribution (undersize)

RESULT: The size distribution of given powder material is from ....to .... μm.

AIM: To determine the particle size distribution by sedimentation method

REFERENCE: Subrahmanyam C.V.S., Textbook of physical pharmaceutics, Vallabh parkashan, 2007, 201-204

APPARATUS: Andreason pipette

CHEMICALS: deflocculating agent, medium

THEORY: Sedimentation method can be used over a size range of 1 -200µm. In this method size is expressed as Stoke's diameter, dst, which describes the diameter of an equivalent sphere having the same rate of sedimentation as that of asymmetric particle. Sedimentation method finds application in

1. formulation and evaluation of suspensions

2. formulation and evaluation of emulsions

3. determination of molecular weight of polymers

Physical stability of a suspension depends on the rate of settling of particles in the dosage form. Similar arguments have been proposed for the evaluation of physical stability of emulsions.

The rate of settling of particle in a suspension or emulsion may be obtained by Stoke's law.

PROCEDURE:

1. Prepare 1 or 2% suspension of the powder in a suitable medium.
2. Add a suitable deflocculating agent which will help in uniform dispersion of the suspension.
3. Transfer the suspension into the andreason vessel. Place the stopper and shake the vessel to distribute the suspension uniformly.

4. Remove the stopper and place the two-way pipette and securely suspend the vessel in a constant temperature water bath.

5. At different time intervals, withdraw 10 ml samples using two way stopcock and collect in a watch glass.

6. Evaporate the samples and weigh. Report the weight or the amount of particles obtained in each time interval as weight undersize.

RESULT: The size distribution of given powder material is from ....to .... μm

AIM: To determine the shelf life of aspirin solution (in 0.1N HCl solution) using accelerated stability studies.

REFERENCE: Subrahmanyam C.V.S., Textbook of physical pharmaceutics, Vallabh parkashan, 2007, 71-75

APPARATUS: Pipettes, volumetric flask (10ml), measuring cylinder ,UV-spectrophotometer ,conical flask, water bath, weighing balance, test-tubes

CHEMICALS REQUIRED: salicylic acid, HCl solution, aspirin powder, ferric nitrate solution, distilled water.

THEORY: Most of the drugs purchased from the retail shop contain expiry date on the label of the pack. The expiry date is an assurance given by the manufacturer, that if the product is taken before the expiry of the labeled date, the dosage fulfils the specifications presented on the label regarding identity, strength, quality and purity. The drug control department ensures through regulatory controls that every product released into the market should be evaluated to fix the expiry date. The technical term for expiry time is shelf-life. Shelf life is defined as the time required for a drug to reduce its concentration to 90 % of the labeled concentration. The evaluation of shelf life is essential because the stability of a drug in dosage forms can be influenced by the normal environmental conditions. Accelerated stability studies are an experimental design to evaluate the stability of a product by accelerating the rate of reaction. The exponential equation is :-

$$K = Ae^{-Ea/RT}$$

Where K= specific rate constant

A= frequency factor or Arrehenius factor

= energy of activation in KJ/mol. K

T= Absolute temperature

Log K= log A- E_a/2303RT

E_a =slope x 2.303Xr

Where R= 8.314J/mol. K (Universal gas constant)

During storage conditions, aspirin undergoes hydrolysis to salicylic acid and acetic acid .Aspirin follows pseudo first order kinetics in the acidic medium.

Procedure: I) Standard curve preparation:-

1. Weigh accurately 100 mg of salicylic acid and transfer in volumetric flask (100ml), make the volume upto the mark with distilled water (Solution A).
2. Pipette 10 ml of solution A into a volumetric flask (100ml) and dilute upto 100ml with distilled water (Solution B).
3. Prepare (4%w/v) ferric nitrate solution by dissolving 4gm ferric nitrate in 100ml of water.
4) From solution B, take different volumes like 0.1ml, 0.2ml, 0.3ml, 0.4ml, 0.5ml, 0.6ml, 0.7ml & 0.8ml , add 1ml of ferric nitrate solution (4%w/v) to each and dilute upto 10ml with distilled water.
5) Measure the absorbance at 547 nm in UV spectrophotometer taking distilled water as blank.
6) Plot the graph between concentration and absorbance.
II) Accelerated stability studies:-
1) Weigh accurately about 100mg of aspirin and transfer into 250ml conical flask.
2) Add 1 or 2 ml of alcohol to dissolve the aspirin and make up to 100ml with HCl solution (0.1N).
3) Cork the conical flask and keep in a water bath at 40 degree celcius.
4) Immediately after placing in water bath, take 1ml of mixture which represents zero time samples.
5) Withdraw 1ml of samples into test-tubes at regular interval of 10, 20,30,40,50 and 60 minutes from the mixture container.
6) Add about 2 ml of ferric nitrate solution to each test tube and make up the volume to 10ml with HCl solution (0.1N)

7) Measure the absorbance at 547nm in UV spectrophotometer against a blank.

8) Plot the graph taking time on X-axis and log percent aspirin undecomposed on Y-axis.

9) Repeat the whole procedure at 60 degree celcius and 70 degree celcius.

Observations:- I) Standard curve of salicylic acid:-

Concentration(μg/ml)	Absorbance
10	
20	
40	
60	
80	
100	

II) Aspirin decomposition at 40^{0}C

Time (min)	Absorbance	Conc. (mg/ml)	Aspirin decomposed (mg/ml) (X)	Aspirin undecomposed (100-X)	%Aspirin undecomposed (100-X)x100	log%aspirin remain undecompoded
0	0.055	0.786	1.022	98.978	9897.8	3.9955
10	0.057	0.82	1.066	98.934	9893.4	3.9953
20	0.060	0.87	1.131	98.869	9886.9	3.9950
30	0.062	0.903	1.173	98.826	9882.6	3.9948
40						
50						
60						

III) Aspirin decomposition at 60°C –Same as above

IV) Aspirin decomposition at 70 degree celcius-Same as above

Calculate the slope from the graph, then calculate log K values. Plot the observed log K values against the reciprocal of absolute temperature (1/T).

From the graph, the log K_{25} was extrapolated.

Log K_{25} = -3.33

K_{25} = 0.00046

Shelf-life at $25^{\circ}C$

= t_{90} = 0.104/ K_{25} = 2.26086 hours = 9.42 days

Substitute the K_{25} value in the equation of an appropriate order to get the shelf –life of the product under normal shelf conditions.

RESULT: The shelf life of aspirin solution as determined by accelerated stability studies is..........days.

AIM: To determine the density of water at different temperature by using specific gravity bottle (pycnometer)

REFERENCE: Indian pharmacopoeia

APPARATUS: Density bottle, weighing balance, thermometer, water-bath, refrigerator, ice-cold water.

Procedure: 1) Take a clean and dry pycnometer and weigh it, let its weight be W_1 gm.

2) Keep the samples of water at different temperatures like refrigerator(4 degree celcius),room temperature(25 degree celcius) and heat the water samples to different temperatures like 30 degree C,40 C,50C,60C.

3) Fill the pycnometer with water (at room temperature), close its lid & wipe the outside with tissue paper and weigh it. Let it be w_2 gm.

4) Calculate the weight (w_3) of water.

$W_3 = w_2 - w_1 \text{gm}$

5) Find the density of water at room temperature.

$P = w_2 - w_1/25 \text{ gm /ml}$

Where 25 means volume of the pycnometer (25ml)

6) Similarly repeat the procedure for the water samples kept at different temperatures.

7) Plot the graph taking temperature on x-axis and density on y-axis.

Observations:

Temperature(^{0}C)	Density(gm/ml)

RESULT: The density of water increases/decreases with the rise in temperature.

AIM: To study the effect of sodium chloride in different concentration on density of water

REFERENCE: Indian pharmacopoeia

Apparatus: specific gravity bottle, weighing balance, tissue paper, volumetric flasks

CHEMICALS: sodium chloride, purified water

Procedure: 1) Prepare sodium chloride solutions (1%,5%, 7.5%, 10%, 20%w/v) by weighing 1g,5g.7.5g,10g,20 g of sodium chloride and dilute upto 100ml with water to prepare respective concentrations.

2) Take a clean pycnometer and weigh it. Let it be W_1gm.

3) Fill the pycnometer with water at room temperature, stopper it and note its weight. Let it be $w_2$gm.

4) Note the weight of water and calculate its density using the formula

$\rho = w_2\text{-}w_1/25$ gm /ml

5) Similarly repeat the procedure for different salt solutions and measure the density.

6) Then plot the graph between concentration on x-axis and density on y-axis.

Observations:

Concentration (%w/v)	Density(gm/ml)
1	
5	
7.5	
10	
20	

Result: The density of water increases/decreases with the increase in concentration of salt.

AIM: To prepare the different concentration of sucrose and determine the density at room temperature

REFERENCE: Indian pharmacopoeia

Requirements: Pycnometer, weighing balance, tissue paper, sucrose, purified water , volumetric flasks(100ml)

Procedure: 1) Take a clean pycnometer and weigh. Let its weight be $w_1$gm.

2) Prepare different concentrations of sucrose solutions by weighing 1g, 5g, 7.5g, 10g & 20g of sucrose and dissolve in water and make up the volume upto 100ml.

3) Fill the pycnometer with water, stopper it , wipe the outside with tissue paper and weigh it .Let it be $w_2$gm.

4) Calculate the density of solutions using the formula:

$\rho = w_2\text{-}w_1/25 \text{ gm }/\text{ml}$

5) Similarly repeat the step 3 for different sucrose solutions and find the density using specific gravity bottles.

6) Finally plot the graph between concentration on x-axis and density on y-axis.

Observations:

Concentration of sucrose Solution(%w/v)	Density(gm/ml)
0	
1	
5	
7.5	
10	
20	

RESULT: The density of water increases/decreases with the rise in concentration of sucrose.

AIM: To prepare 100ml of a pharmaceutical buffer of pH 5.0(acetate buffer) and verify the same by measuring pH using pH meter.

Reference: Indian pharmacopoeia

Requirements: Weighing balance, volumetric flask (100ml), pH meter, sodium acetate, glacial acetic acid, purified water

Procedure: Preparation of acetate buffer (pH 5.0)

1) Weigh 1.36 gm of sodium acetate and transfer into a 100ml volumetric flask, add 0.6ml of glacial acetic acid and add sufficient water to produce 100ml.
2) Calibrate the pH meter with standard buffer solutions of pH 4.0 & pH 7.0
3) Transferred the prepared acetate buffer (pH 5.0) into a beaker and measure its pH with the pH meter.
4) Adjust the pH with sodium hydroxide solution or hydrochloric solution if not proper.

    RESULT: The buffer of ...... pH was prepared and verified using calibrated pH meter.

AIM: To study the effect of concentration on surface tension

REFERENCE: Subrahmanyam C.V.S., Textbook of physical pharmaceutics, Vallabh parkashan, 2007, 132-133

Apparatus: Stalagmometer, rubber tube, burette stand, volumetric flask, weighing balance, beakers, stopwatch.

Chemicals: sodium lauryl sulphate, purified water

Theory: Surface tension is defined as the force in dynes acting on a surface at right angle to any line of unit length or per cm.

There are two methods of determining surface tension.

1. Drop weight method

2. Drop number method

Surface tension of a liquid is measured by using an apparatus called stalagmometer. This method is based on the principle that the weight of liquid falling from a capillary tube held vertical is approximately proportional to the surface of the liquid. It is more convenient to count the number of drops of the liquid than finding the weight of a single drop. The weights of equal volumes of two liquids are proportional to their densities. If n_1 and n_2 are the number of drops of two liquids of the same volume, then

$$Y_1/Y_2 = n_2 d_1 / n_1 d_2$$

Where Y_1 and Y_2 are surface tensions of water and solution respectively.

Stalagmometer is used for relative methods of determination of surface tension of liquids. It consists of a capillary tube the end of which is flattened to provide a large dropping surface with a sharp boundary. The capillary tube extends upwards into bulb which terminates again into a capillary on either ends of bulb are found marks X and Y the surface tension may be determined by counting of drops formed by liquid volume from X and Y. The number of drops is counted for a liquid provided with a scale the fraction of the drop may be estimated to an accuracy of 0.05 of a drop. To check the flow the capillary tube is attached to a rubber tube filled with a pinch cork at one of the ends the rate of flow should not exceed 15 drops/minute if it is more than this it should be decreased with the help of rubber tube with pinch cork.

Procedure:

1) Take a clean and dry stalagmometer
2) Suck distilled water into the stalagmometer till the level reaches to the top mark above the bulb X.
3) Now allow the water to flow through the capillary and count the number of drops fallen till the level reaches the lowest mark below the bulb Y.
4) Prepare 2 % detergent solution by dissolving 2gm of sodium lauryl sulphate in a100ml distilled water in 100ml volumetric flask.
5) Repeat steps 2 and 3 with 2 % surfactant solution and find the number of drops.
6) Transfer 50 ml of the 2 % solution into 100ml volumetric flask and dilute upto 100ml with water to prepare 1 % solution.
7) Repeat the steps 2 &3 with 1% solution.
8) Transfer 50 ml of 1% solution into a clean volumetric flask (100ml) and dilute upto 100ml with water to prepare 0.5 % solution and find the surface tension.
9) Further transfer 50 ml of 0.5 % solution and dilute upto 100ml with water to prepare 0.25 % solution & repeat steps 2 and 3.
   10) Take 50 ml of 0.25 % solution % dilute upto 100ml with water to prepare 0.125 % solution and find the surface tension.
   11) Find the surface tension of each solution using the formula:

$$Y_2 = n_2 d_1 / n_1 d_2 \times Y_1$$

Where n_1= number of drops of water between the marks X and Y

n_2 = number of drops of given solution between the marks

d_1 = density of water at room temperature

d_2= density of given liquid

Y_1= surface tension of water (72dyne/cm)

Y_2= surface tension of given solution at room temperature

Density of each solution can be found using pycnometer (specific gravity bottle)

12) Record the data in table and plot the graph between concentration on x-axis and surface tension on y-axis.

Observations:

S. No.	Solution	Conc. of solution(%w/v)	Number of drops	Surface tension(dynes/cm)
1	Water	0		72
2	SLS solution	2		
3	SLS sol.	1		
4	SLS sol.	0.5		
5	SLS sol.	0.25		
6	SLS sol.	0.125		

Result: The surface tension of water increases/decreases with the increase in concentration of sodium lauryl sulphate (surfactant) in water.

AIM: To determine the HLB value of the given material (glyceryl monostearate) by saponification method

Reference: physical pharmacy-Martin

Method: determine the saponification value of the given substance using I.P. method.

APPARATUS: Weighing balance, measuring cylinder, round bottomed flask, reflux condenser, water bath, burette, burette stand

CHEMICALS: Potassium hydroxide, purified water, glyceryl monostearate, HCl, alcohol, Tween 20, sodium carbonate, methyl orange indicator

Theory: Saponification number is the amount of potassium hydroxide required to neutralize the fatty acids, resulting from the complete hydrolysis of 1 gram of oil or fat when determined by the following method (I.P. 66, Page 936).

Procedure:

1) Weigh about 35-40 gram of potassium hydroxide and dissolve in 20 ml of water and add sufficient alcohol to make 1000ml.Allow it to stand overnight and pour off the clear liquid.

2)Weigh accurately about 2 gram of given substance (glyceryl monostearate) in a tared 250 ml round bottomed flask, add 25 ml of alcoholic KOH solution ,attach a reflux condenser and boil in a water bath for one hour frequently rotating the contents of the flask, cool and add 1ml of phenolphthalein solution and add titrate the excess of alkali with 0.5 N HCl. Note the number of ml consumed=a ml. Repeat the experiment with same reagents in the same manner omitting the given substance which is treated as blank. Note the number of ml required = b ml.

3) Calculate saponification value using the following formula:

Saponification number= (b-a) x 0.02805x1000/w

w = weight of given substance in grams

Polyoxyethylene sorbitan monolaurate (Tween 20)

S=45.5

A =276(Acid value of lauric acid)

HLB=16.7

Glyceryl monostearate

S= 170(approx)

A= 197(acid value of stearic acid)

HLB =3.8

Preparation & standardization of 0.5N HCl

Dilute 20 times 10 N solution of HCl (1 part HCl +19 part water) prepare 250 ml.

Standardise using sodium carbonate AR using methyl orange as indicator.

Normality=weight x 1000/eq. weight (153)x volume

W=200-300mg approx.

RESULT: The HLB value of given material was found to be............

AIM: To determine the sedimentation volume of the suspensions using different suspending agents

---

References:

1) More HN, Hazare AA, Practical physical pharmacy. Career publications,2010:203-205
2) Gaud RS, Gupta GD. Practical physical pharmacy, CBS Publisher and distributor, 2009: 81-84.
3) Mohanta GP, Physical pharmacy, practical text, pharma book syndicate, 2006: 72-74.

APPARATUS: mortar & pestle, weighing balance, spatula, measuring cylinder, ruler

Chemicals: calamine, acacia gum, tragacanth gum, bentonite, purified water

Theory: A suspension is a heterogenous system containing solids dispersed in the vehicle in such a size that they do not settle down. Wheather a pharmaceutical suspension is to be taken orally, applied topically or injected, the dispersed phase should be uniformly distributed in order to ensure the administration of a uniform dose. The rate of sedimentation or settling for a suspended phase depends on several factors which are under the control of the formulator or pharmacist. Stokes developed an equation which related the rate of sedimentation to the physical properties of the suspension known as stoke's law as given below:

$$\frac{dx}{dt} = 2r^2(\rho_1 - \rho_2)g/9x\eta$$

where r is the radius of the dispersed phase,

ρ_1 is the density of the particles, ρ_2 is the density of medium (vehicle) & g is the gravitational constant. η is the viscosity of the medium.

Although the stoke's law does not consider all variables which affect a suspension, it gives an approximation of the rate of settling and an appreciation of the effect which controllable factors exert on the settling rate. By reducing particle size, by increasing viscosity and by increasing the viscosity and by increasing the density of the external phase, we can retard the sedimentation rate.

Suspending agents are physiologically inert substances which increase viscosity when added to the suspensions. On prolonged standing , suspensions tend to cake by crystal formation at the bottom of container. Therefore, a second important function for suspending agents is to facilitate redistribution of a suspension on shaking. That is redispersion should be easy. Particles in suspension can come together to form either floccules or aggregates. Floccules form when weak vander walls forces are holding the particles together. Floccules are easy to break apart. However, the large fluffy clumps that characterize a flocculated system settle rapidly. It is the goal of the good formulator to develop a system which controls the rate of flocculation and sedimentation.

Procedure:

1) Take a clear four 100 ml graduated cylinders
2) Take a four mortar & pestle and clean them
3) To the first, add preweighed 5gm of calamine. Add the water slowly and triturate until a smooth paste is formed.
4) To the second mortar, add 5 gm of calamine and 2 gm of preweighed acacia gum, triturate until a smooth paste is formed.
5) To the third mortar, add 5 gm of calamine and 2 gm of weighed bentonite.
6) To the fourth mortar, add 5 gm of calamine and add 1 gm of tragacanth gum.
7) Add some rinsing water to each mortar, transfer the contents of the mortar to the graduated 100 ml measuring cylinders, rinse the mortar with additional water and add the rinsing to the measuring cylinder. Make up the volume upto 100ml with water quantity sufficient. Keep the suspension on shelf (flat surface) undisturbed. Record the appearance of suspension (fine ,turbid etc) and volume of the sediment formed (height) at 5 min,15min,45min and 90 min. Prepare an observation table and plot the results and compare the suspending efficiency of different suspending agents. The suspension which contains minimum height of sediment is better

suspension and is better suspending agent. Evaluate different suspending agents. Prepare a bar graph for different suspending agents . Plot the graph between sedimentation volume & time for different suspending agents.

RESULT: The suspension prepared by ....suspending agent showed minimum sedimentation volume with time hence this suspending agent is best.

AIM: To prepare a flocculating and deflocculating suspension of magnesium carbonate and assess their stability.

REFERENCE: Subrahmanyam C.V.S., Textbook of physical pharmaceutics, Vallabh parkashan, 2007, 369-372

APPARATUS: mortar & pestle, measuring cylinder, rular

Chemicals: Magnesium carbonate, Aluminium chloride

Theory: Magnesium carbonate is an insoluble but diffusible solid. In flocculated suspension, the particles settle more quickly than particles of deflocculating one. But the sediment form a hard cake in deflocculated suspension making redispersibility on shaking difficult. Hence comparing the two types of suspension, the flocculated one is pharmaceutically acceptable or preferable due to elegant appearance, however a controlled flocculation is desirable to achieve a controlled sedimentation with ease of dispersibility. Electrolytes and ionic surfactants can be used as flocculating agents to produce a flocculated suspension. Suspensions without floculating agent is a deflocculated one. Floculated agents (Ionic surfactants) act by neutralizing the charge on each particle, resulting into a flocculated suspension. When the surfactants reduce the interfacial tension, the liquid becomes capable of displacing the absorbed film of air from the surface of solid drug particle and facilitate wetting. The flocculating agents act by shrinkage of ionic double layer or neutralizing the surface charge of suspended particles or bridging between particles.

Procedure:I Preparation of deflocculated suspension

1) Take a clean mortar and powdered the light magnesium carbonate(5gm)
2) Add water slowly to the mortar alongwith trituration until a smooth cream /paste is formed. Dilute it sufficiently with water.

3) Then transfer to a graduated measuring cylinder. Reapeatedly rinse the mortar with little water every time and the rinsed mixture subsequently to adjust the volume to 100ml.

II Preparation of flocullated suspension

1) Take a clean mortar and add light magnesium carbonate(5gm)
2) Dissolve small quantity of aluminium chloride in little water and add this solution to mortar with trituration until a smooth cream is formed .Transfer the cream to the measuring cylinder after dilution with water.
3) Repeatedly rinse the mortar with little amount of water every time and add the rinsed mixture subsequently to adjust the volume.

III: 1) Thoroughly shake the cylinders to make the suspensions uniform

2) Keep the cylinders undisturbed on a flat surface after shaking.

3) Note the volume (height) of sediment formed at different time intervals i.e. 0,10,30,45 & 60 minutes in the case of both suspensions.

Original volume of suspension = 100ml = V_0 = volume at 0 minutes

Volume at 10 minutes V_1 =

Volume at 30 minutes V_2 =

Volume at 45 minutes V_3 =

Volume at 60 minutes V_4 =

The degree of flocculation at one hour = sediment volume of flocculated suspension in one hour/sediment volume of deflocculated sediment in one hour

Plot the sedimentation volume on Y-axis and time on X-axis

(Sedimentation volume quickly decrease in flocculated suspension compared to deflocculated suspension initially but ultimate sedimentation volume of flocculated will be higher.

Observation table:

Time in minutes	Vol. of sediment for flocculated suspension in ml	Sedimentation volume in deflocculated suspension
0		
10		
30		
45		
60		

Result: Write about which suspension (flocculated or deflocculated) showed better results